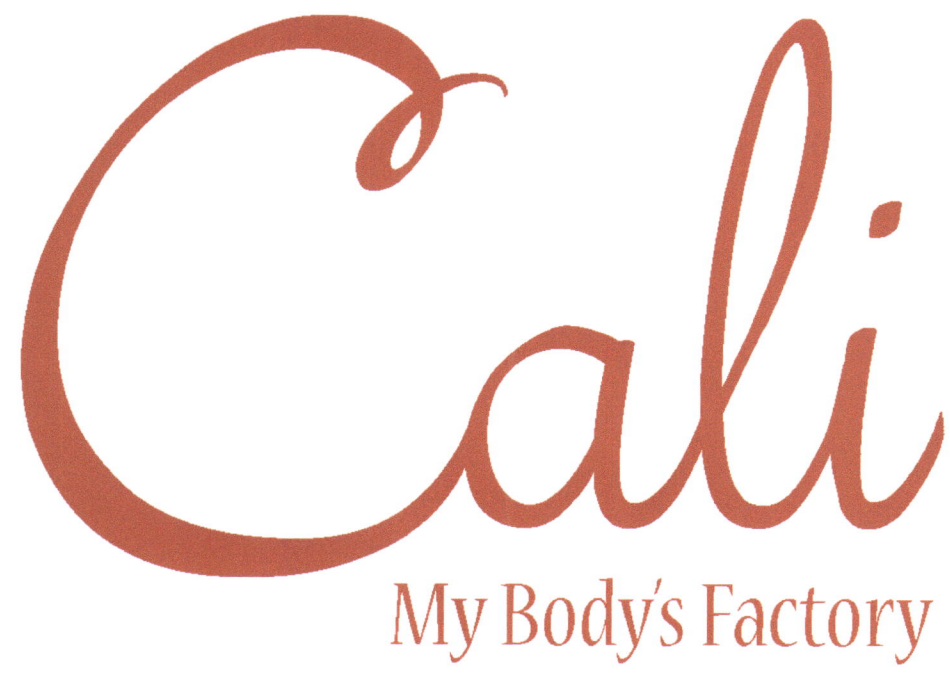

Cali

My Body's Factory

Written by: Nancy Otis Alber  Illustrated by: Kristin Hone Schieterman

ISBN: 153008380X
ISBN 13: 9781530083800

Library of Congress Control Number: 2016910034
CreateSpace Independent Publishing Platform, North Charleston, SC

To my sweet Cali, my inspiration
To my dearest Aunt Patty, my lifetime admiration
To my dear husband Harold, for your unflagging love and support

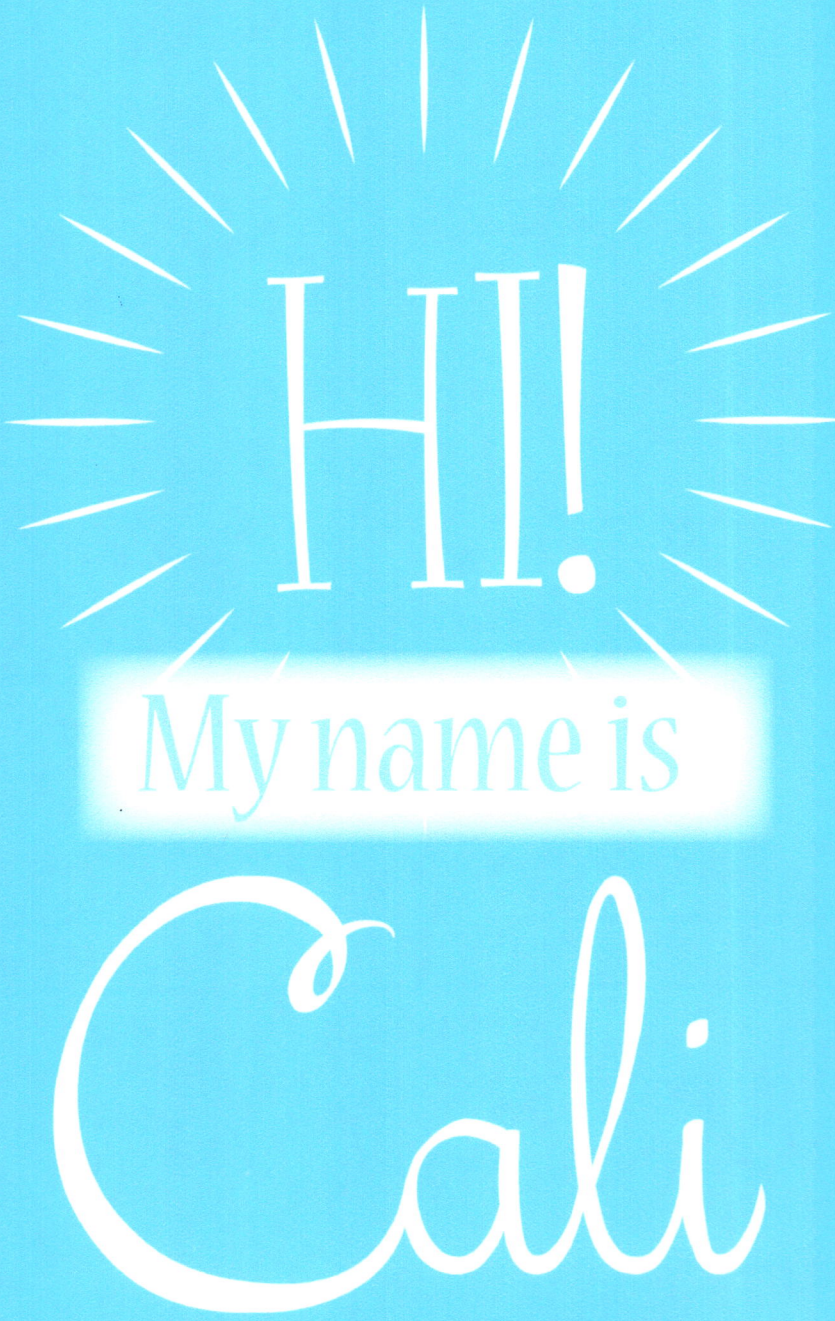

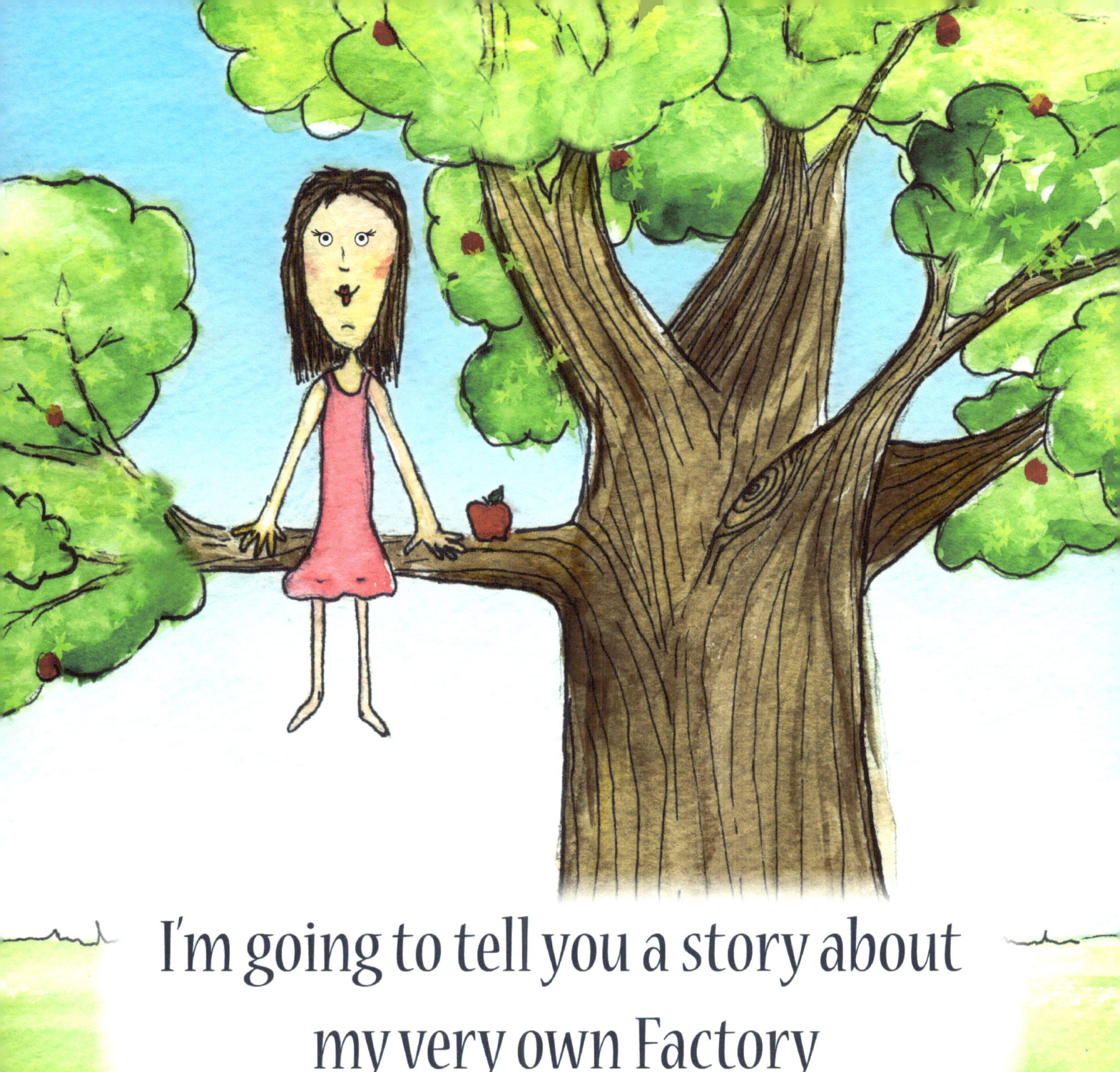

I'm going to tell you a story about my very own Factory

My dad's name is

Lloyd

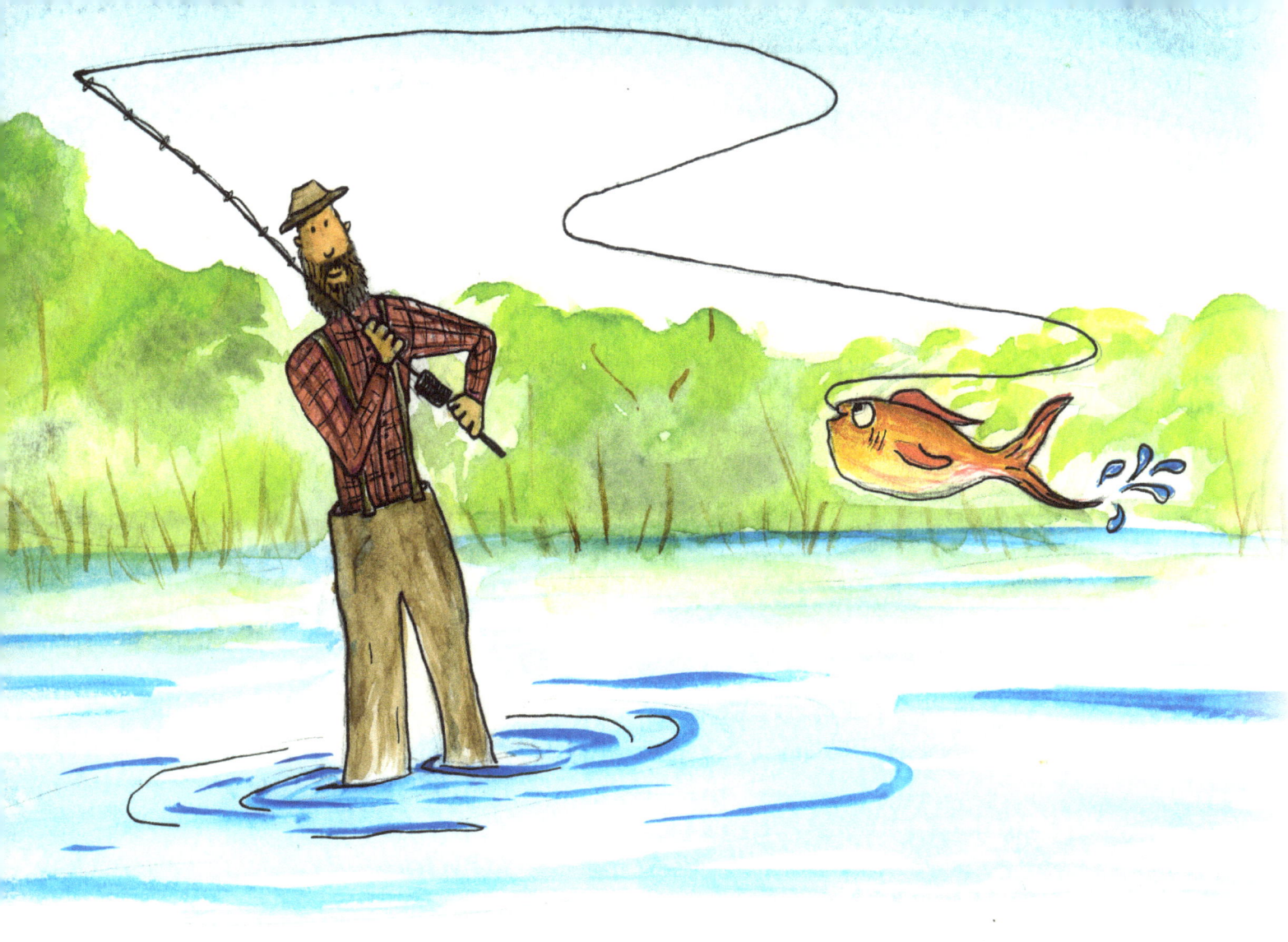

He's a doctor who's a strong guy and likes to fish.
Dad is catching our dinner

My mom's name is

Alice

She takes care of our garden and cooks our food!

I sometimes have to weed our garden, *which I don't like*

But I do it because mom says so and the weeds will choke and hurt the other plants. I do like climbing trees to *pick apples for dessert*

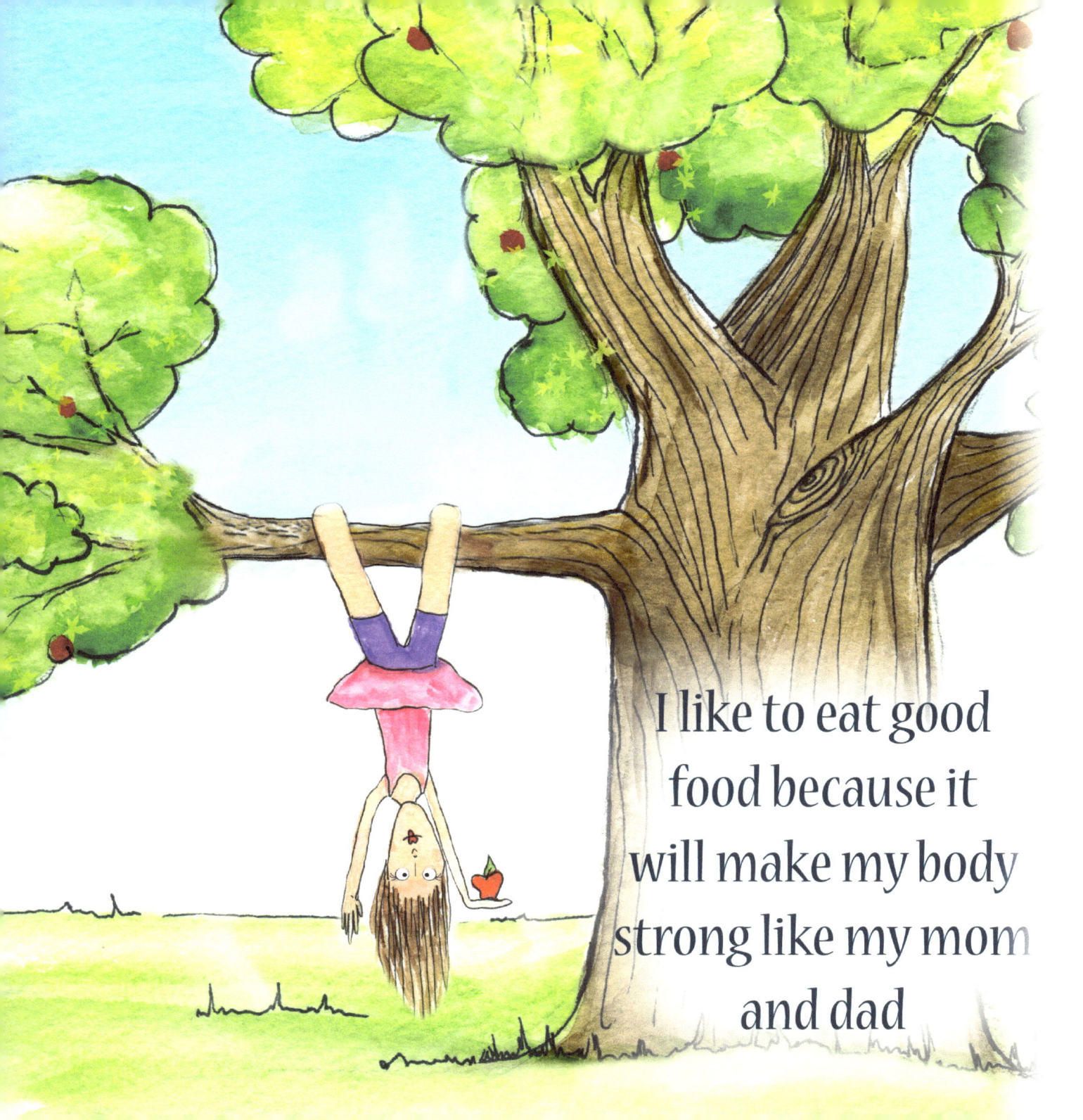

I like to eat good
food because it
will make my body
strong like my mom
and dad

My body is like a factory. My mouth is the entry door of my factory. My stomach is the food prep part fo my factory. The food I eat goes into my stomach where it gets all ground up so it can *move on to my intestines.* My upper intestines are the precessing part of my factory. It separates the *good part* of my food from the garbage part.

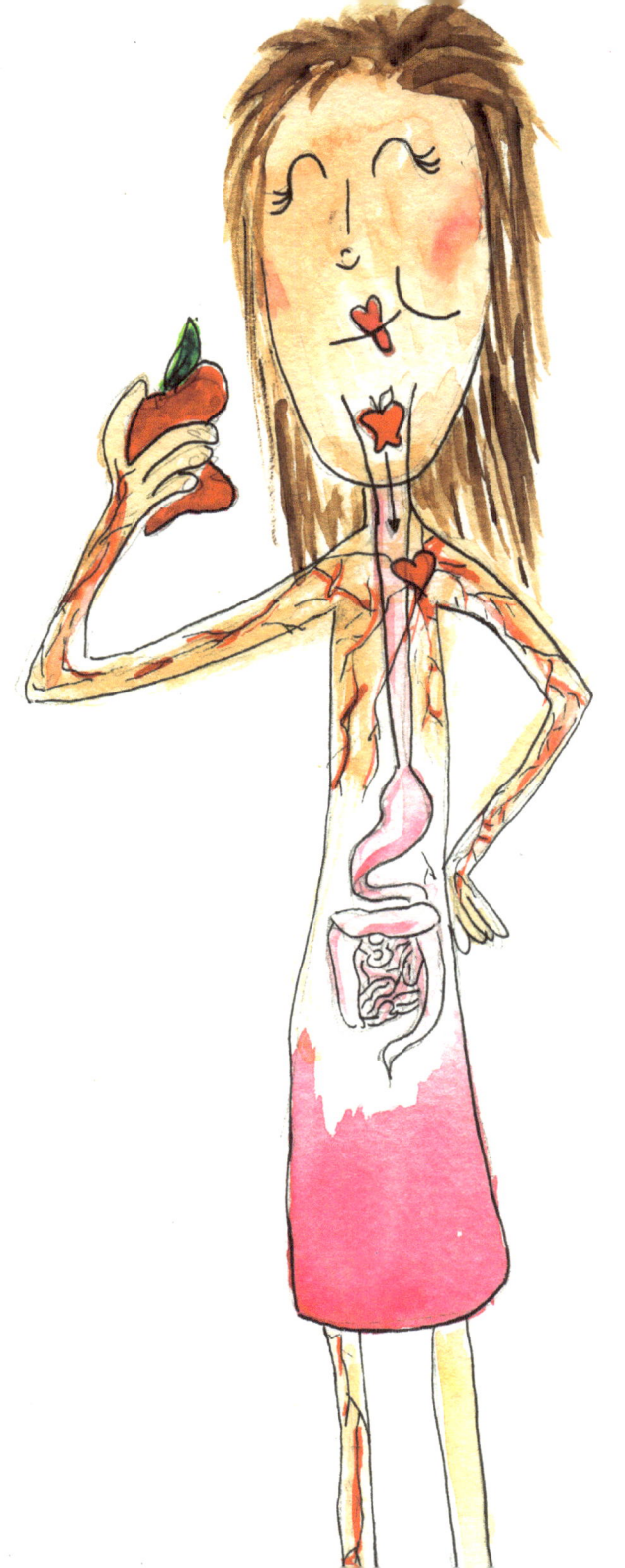

The good part goes from my intestines to the transportation part of my factory (my blood stream) where it travels all over nourshing my body so it can get strong.

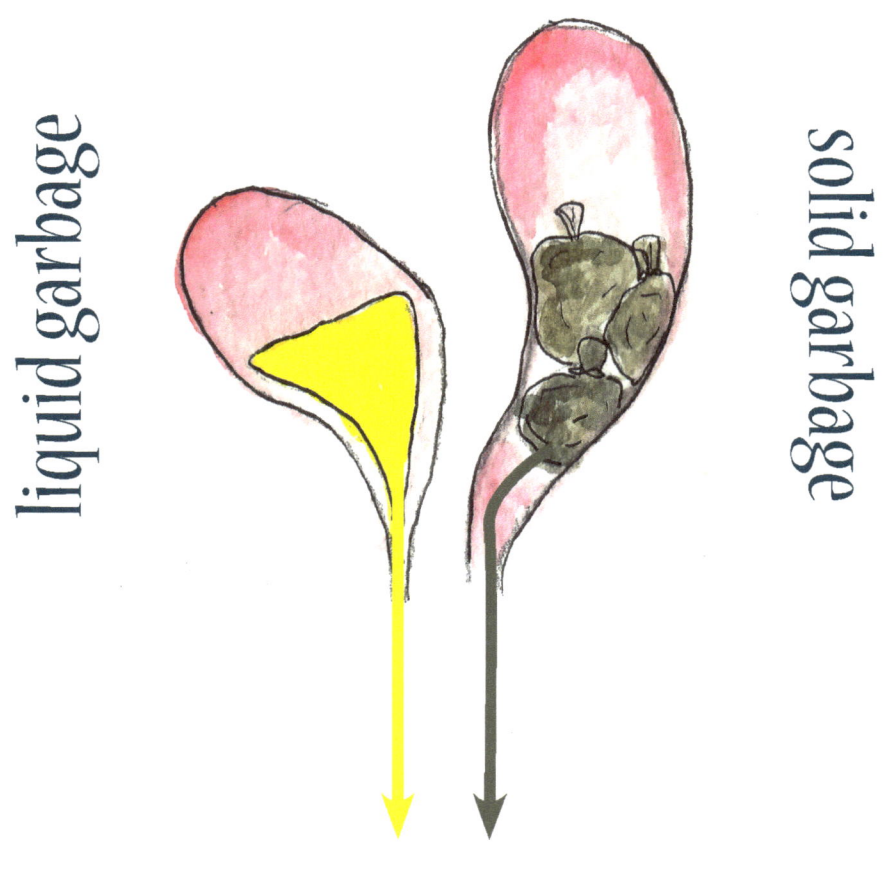

liquid garbage

solid garbage

Exits the body

The part of my food that is not needed to feed my body goes to the garbage department of my factory.
The liquid part moves on to my bladder and the solid part moves to my lower intestines.
Here the stuff sits until I enpty the garbage

Because I'm a big girl and no longer wear diapers, I go to the toilet to get rid of the garbage

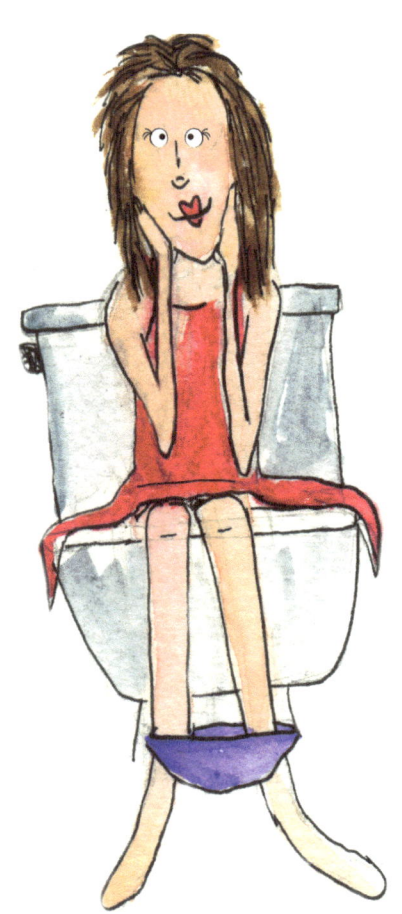

It's *very important* that I go to the toilet and get rid of that garbage in my body, or it just

keeps filling up my garbage compartments and

filling them up and filling them up

until they get so full bad things happen.

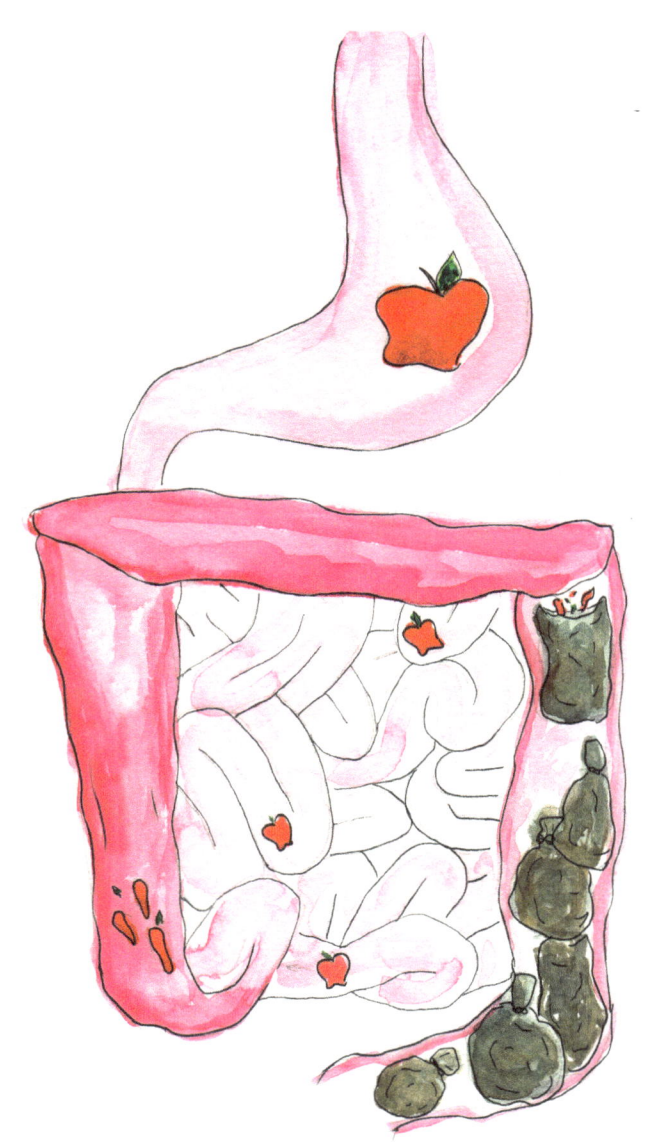

The bladder, the liquid garbage department would get so full that i could wet myself so that

everybody would think I'm a baby again

or even worse,

it would get so full it would start sucking the bad stuff back into my body

which would make me very sick.

If the solid garbage departmetn gets too full it starts getting so crammed up that it gets very hard

inside so that it won't come out and thatt makes a big prolem for me. So instead of my factory making

me strong, so I can climb trees, run, and play, it would make me sick and weak

and that's not good!

So take my advice and eats lots of good food to make your factory as strong and empty your garbage departments on a regular basis!

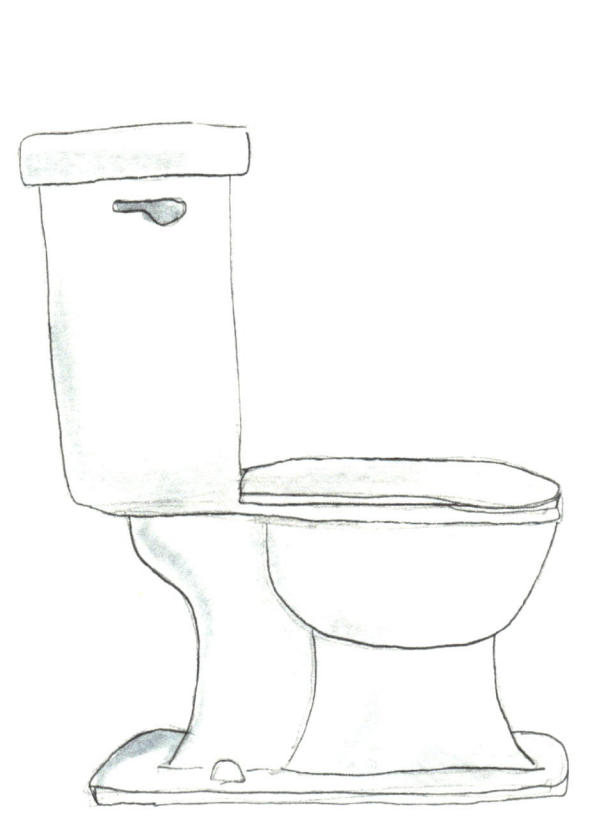
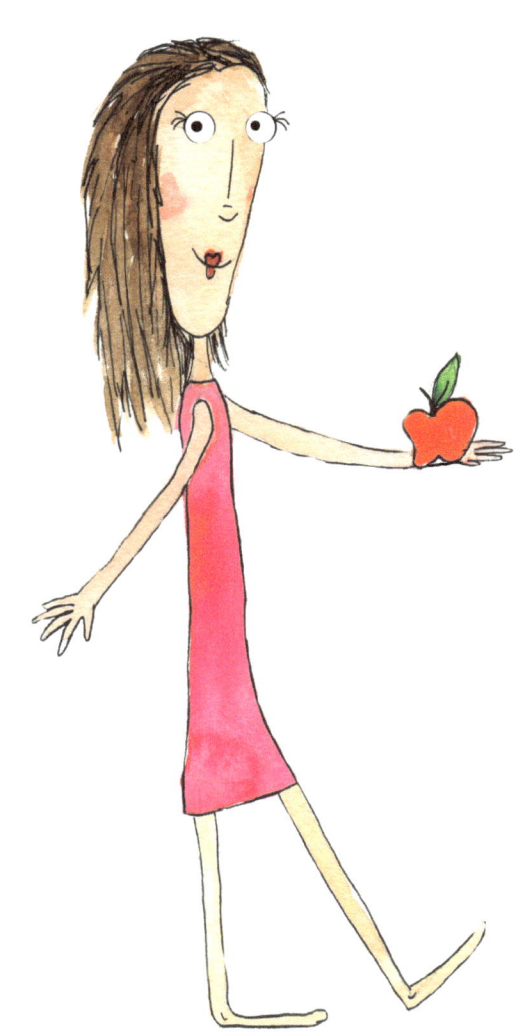